The Complete Med Dinner Cook

Tasty and Healthy Dinner Recipes to Start Your Mediterranean Diet and Stay Fit

Carl Ewing

Table of Contents

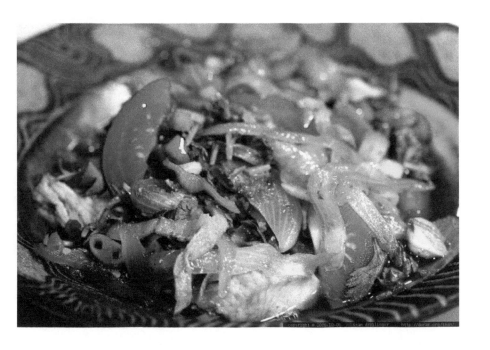

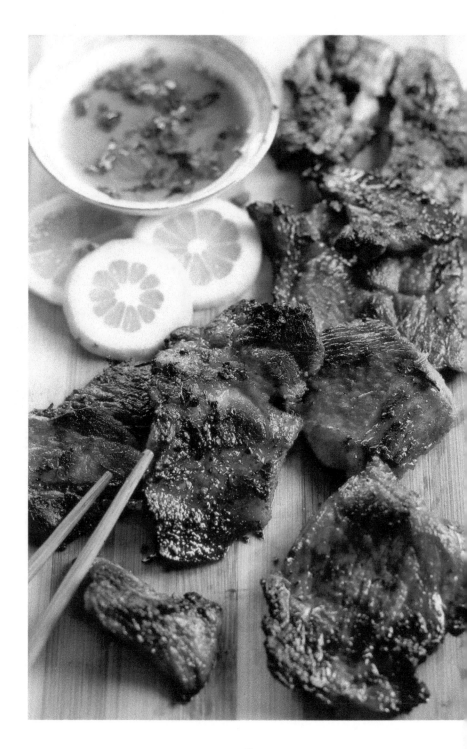

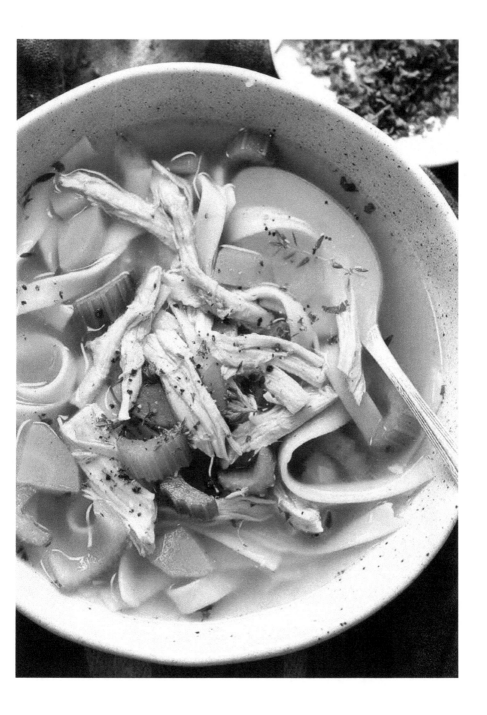

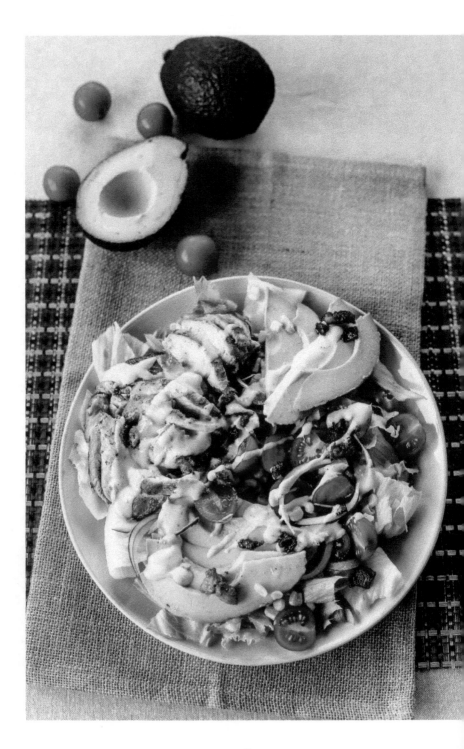

Tomato Soup

Prep time: 5 minutes I **Cooking time:** 25 minutes I
Servings: 4

Ingredients:

- 1 yellow onion, chopped
- 2 tablespoons olive oil
- 2 garlic cloves, minced
- 1 pound tomatoes, cubed
- 2 teaspoons turmeric powder
- ¼ teaspoon cardamom powder
- 5 cups veggie stock
- A pinch of salt and black pepper
- 6 ounces baby spinach
- 2 teaspoons lime juice

Directions:

1. Heat up a pot with the oil over medium heat, add the onion and the garlic and sauté for 5 minutes.
2. Add the tomatoes and the other ingredients, toss, simmer over medium heat for 20 minutes more, ladle into bowls and serve.

Nutrition facts per serving: calories 123, fat 10.1, fiber 3.3, carbs 13.3, protein 2.8

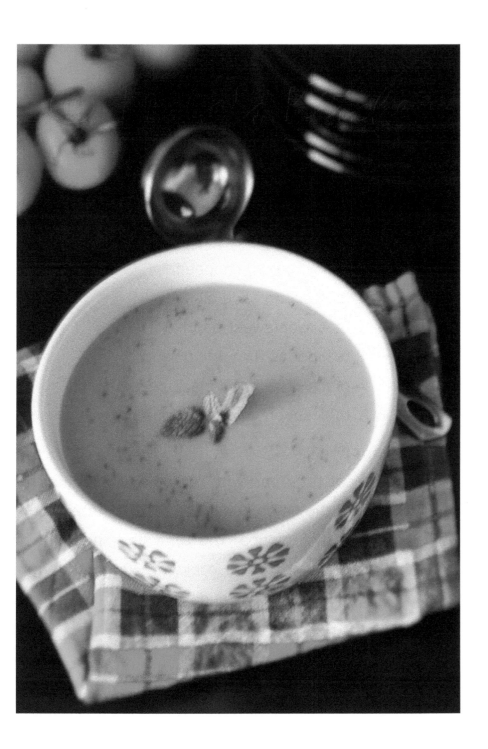

Tuna Bowls

Prep time: 10 minutes I **Cooking time:** 25 minutes I

Servings: 4

Ingredients:

- 2 cups quinoa, cooked
- ½ cup tomato puree
- 3 ounces smoked tuna, boneless and flaked
- 1 yellow onion, chopped
- 1 tablespoon olive oil
- 1 teaspoon sweet paprika
- 2 teaspoons turmeric powder
- A pinch of salt and black pepper
- 1 tablespoon chives, chopped

Directions:

1. Heat up a pan with the oil over medium heat add the onion and sauté for 5 minutes.
2. Add the quinoa, the tuna and the remaining ingredients, toss, cook for 20 minutes more divide into bowls and serve.

Nutrition facts per serving: calories 411, fat 10.7 fiber 7.6, carbs 61, protein 18.7

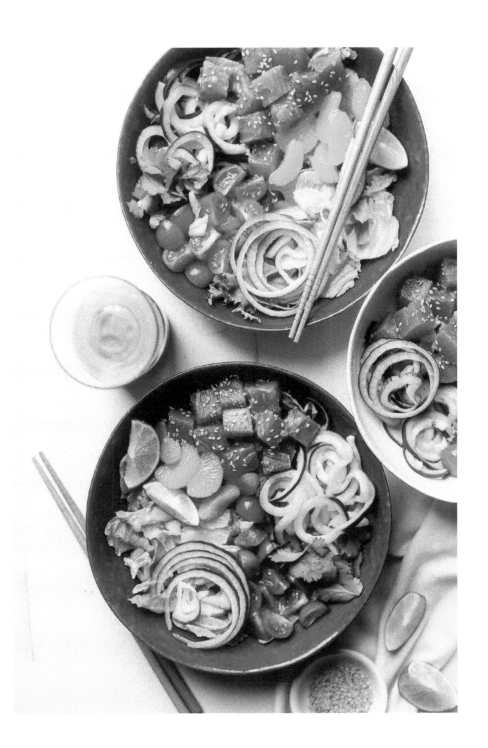

Lemon Trout Mix

Prep time: 5 minutes I **Cooking time:** 25 minutes I

Servings: 4

Ingredients:

- 4 trout fillets, boneless
- 2 scallions, chopped
- 1 cup cauliflower florets
- 2 tablespoons avocado oil
- 2 garlic cloves, minced
- A pinch of salt and black pepper
- Juice of ½ lemon

Directions:

1. In a roasting pan, combine the trout fillets with the scallions and the other ingredients, and bake at 360 degrees F for 25 minutes.
2. Divide the whole mix between plates and serve

Nutrition facts per serving: calories 141, fat 6.3, fiber 1.2, carbs 3, protein 17.4

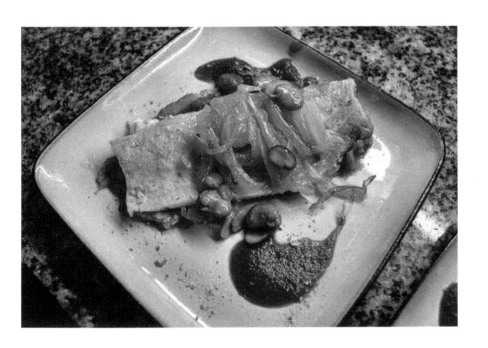

Rosemary Lime Chicken

Prep time: 10 minutes I **Cooking time:** 45 minutes I

Servings: 4

Ingredients:

- 2 chicken breasts, skinless, boneless and halved
- 2 shallots, chopped
- 2 garlic cloves, minced
- 2 tablespoons olive oil
- 1 tablespoon lime juice
- 1 tablespoon parsley, chopped
- 1 tablespoon rosemary, chopped
- 1 tablespoon basil, chopped

Directions:

1. In a roasting pan, combine the chicken breasts with the garlic, shallots and the other ingredients, toss gently and bake at 360 degrees F for 45 minutes.
2. Divide the whole mix between plates and serve for lunch.

Nutrition facts per serving: calories 202, fat 12.4, fiber 0.4, carbs 2, protein 20.6

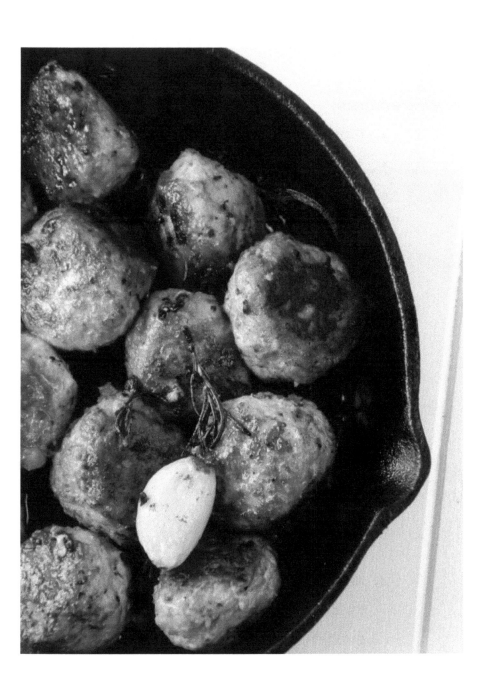

Trout and Asparagus

Prep time: 5 minutes I **Cooking time:** 20 minutes I
Servings: 4

Ingredients:

- 4 trout fillets, boneless
- 1 yellow onion, chopped
- 2 tablespoons olive oil
- 1 bunch asparagus, halved and trimmed
- 3 tablespoons balsamic vinegar
- 1 tablespoon mustard
- 1 garlic clove, minced
- 1 tablespoon chives, chopped
- A pinch of salt and black pepper

Directions:

1. Heat up a pan with the oil over medium-high heat, add the onion and the asparagus and sauté for 3 minutes.
2. Add the fish and sear it for 2 minutes on each side.
3. Add the remaining ingredients, bake everything in the oven at 360 for 13 minutes more, divide everything between plates and serve for lunch

Nutrition facts per serving: calories 266, fat 11, fiber 6, carbs 14.2, protein 9

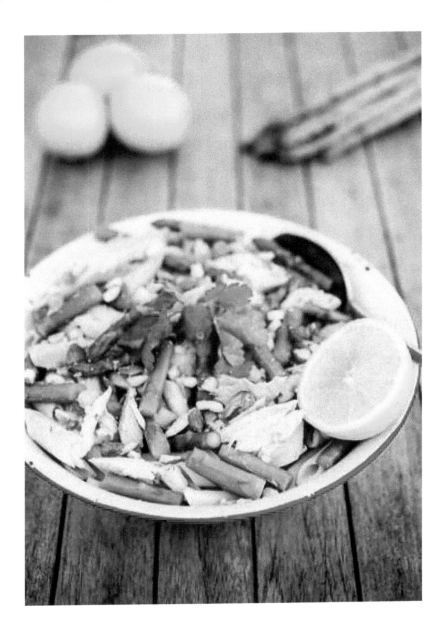

Shrimp Bowls

Prep time: 10 minutes I **Cooking time:** 20 minutes I

Servings: 4

Ingredients:

- 1 yellow onion, chopped
- 1 tablespoon olive oil
- 1 pound shrimp, peeled and deveined
- 1 cup mushrooms, sliced
- ½ cup chicken stock
- A pinch of salt and black pepper
- 1 teaspoon turmeric powder
- 1 tablespoon oregano, chopped

Directions:

1. Heat up a pan with the oil over medium heat add the onion and the mushrooms, stir and sauté for 10 minutes.
2. Add the shrimp and the other ingredients, toss cook everything for 10 minutes more, divide into bowls and serve.

Nutrition facts per serving: calories 261, fat 7, fibe 8, carbs 8.6, protein 7.1

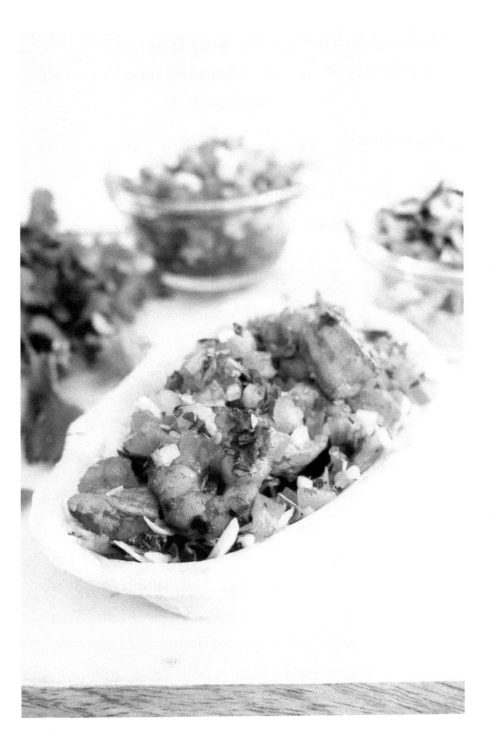

Shrimp with Parsley and Quinoa

Prep time: 5 minutes I **Cooking time:** 10 minutes I

Servings: 4

Ingredients:

- 2 garlic cloves, peeled
- 1 yellow onion, chopped
- 1 pound shrimp, peeled and deveined
- 1 tablespoon olive oil
- 1 cup cherry tomatoes, cut into quarters
- 2 cups quinoa, cooked
- 1 tablespoon parsley, chopped
- 1 teaspoon turmeric powder
- A pinch of salt and black pepper
- A pinch of cayenne pepper

Directions:

1. Heat up a pan with the oil over medium-high heat, add the onion and the garlic and sauté for 2 minutes.
2. Add the tomatoes and sauté for 3 minutes more.
3. Add the shrimp, the quinoa and the rest of the ingredients, toss, cook for 5 minutes more, divide into bowls and serve.

Nutrition facts per serving: calories 261, fat 4, fiber 7, carbs 15, protein 7

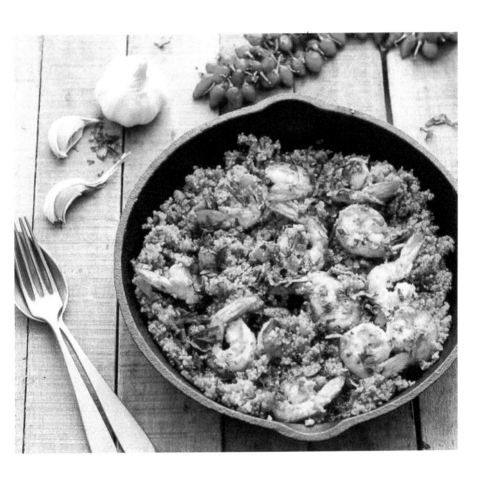

Garlic Chicken Mix

Prep time: 10 minutes I **Cooking time:** 40 minutes I

Servings: 4

Ingredients:

- 2 sweet potatoes, peeled and cut into wedges
- 1 pound chicken breast, skinless, boneless and sliced
- 2 tablespoons olive oil
- 2 scallions, chopped
- A pinch of salt and black pepper
- 2 garlic cloves, minced
- Juice of 1 lime
- ½ cup chicken stock

Directions:

1. In a roasting pan, combine the chicken with the sweet potatoes, the oil and the other ingredients, toss gently and cook at 360 degrees F for 40 minutes.
2. Divide the mix between plates and serve.

Nutrition facts per serving: calories 222, fat 6, fiber 7, carbs 15, protein 7

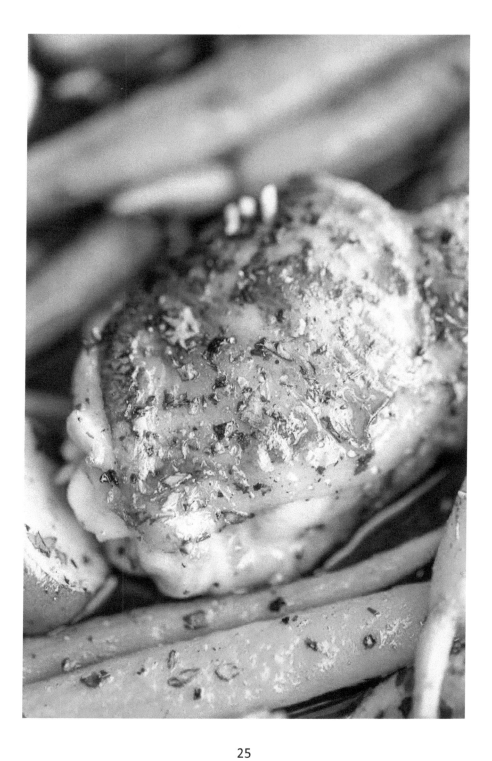

Spiced Chicken Soup

Prep time: 10 minutes I **Cooking time:** 1 hour I

Servings: 8

Ingredients:

- 1 yellow onion, chopped
- 1 pound chicken breast, skinless, boneless and cubed
- 1 tablespoon olive oil
- 2 carrots, sliced
- 3 garlic cloves, minced
- A pinch of salt and black pepper
- 6 cups veggie stock
- 2 teaspoons turmeric powder
- Juice of 1 lime
- Zest of 1 lime, grated
- 1 tablespoon cilantro, chopped

Directions:

1. Heat up a pot with the oil over medium heat, add the onion, carrots and the garlic and sauté for 5 minutes.
2. Add the meat and brown it for 5 minutes more.
3. Add the stock and the other ingredients except the cilantro, toss, bring to a simmer and cook over medium heat for 50 minutes.

4. Divide the soup into bowls, sprinkle the cilantro on top and serve.

Nutrition facts per serving: calories 271, fat 8, fiber 11, carbs 16, protein 8

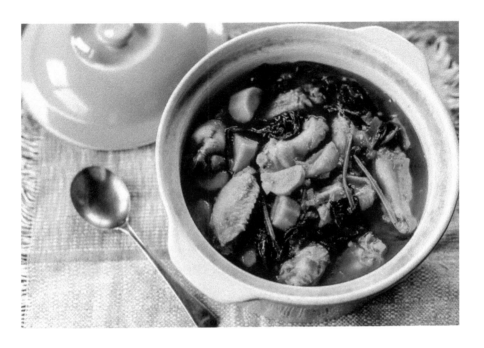

Spinach and Tomato Soup

Prep time: 10 minutes I **Cooking time:** 20 minutes I

Servings: 4

Ingredients:

- 1 pound spinach leaves
- 1 yellow onion, chopped
- 1 tablespoon olive oil
- 4 cups chicken stock
- 4 cherry tomatoes, halved
- 1 red bell pepper, chopped
- 1 tablespoon parsley, chopped

Directions:

1. Heat up a pot with the oil over medium-high heat, add the onion and the bell pepper and sauté for 5 minutes.
2. Add the spinach and the other ingredients, toss, bring to a simmer and cook over medium heat for 15 minutes.
3. Ladle the soup into bowls and serve for lunch.

Nutrition facts per serving: calories 148, fat 2, fiber 6, carbs 8, protein 5

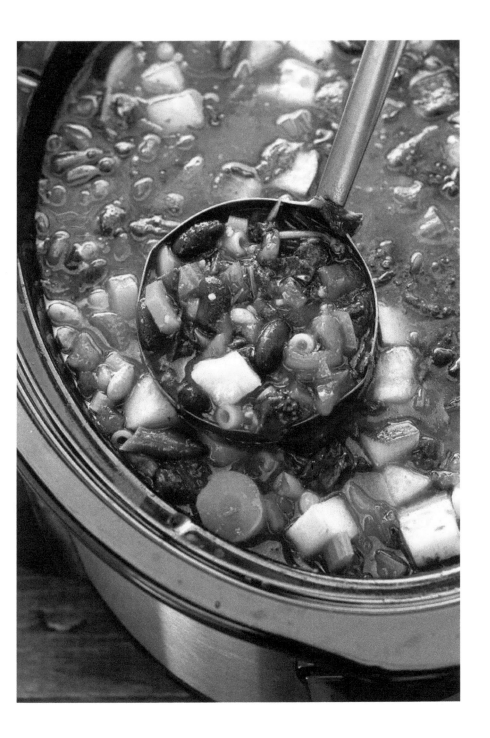

Turkey Meatballs

Prep time: 10 minutes I **Cooking time:** 10 minutes I

Servings: 4

Ingredients:

- 1 pound turkey meat, ground
- 1 yellow onion, chopped
- 1 egg, whisked
- 1 tablespoon cilantro, chopped
- 2 tablespoons olive oil
- 1 red chili pepper, minced
- 2 teaspoons lime juice
- Zest of 1 lime, grated
- A pinch of salt and black pepper
- 1 teaspoon turmeric powder

Directions:

1. In a bowl, combine the turkey meat with the onion and the other ingredients except the oil stir and shape medium meatballs out of this mix.

2. Heat up a pan with the oil over medium-high heat, add the meatballs, cook them for 5 minutes on each side, divide between plates and serve for lunch.

Nutrition facts per serving: calories 200, fat 12, fiber 5, carbs 12, protein 7

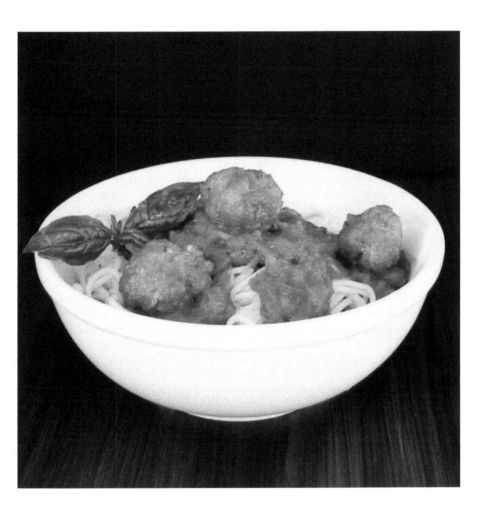

Cauliflower and Tomato Soup

Prep time: 10 minutes I **Cooking time:** 35 minutes I

Servings: 4

Ingredients:

- 1 yellow onion, chopped
- 1 carrot, chopped
- ½ cup celery, chopped
- 1 tablespoon olive oil
- 1 pound cauliflower florets
- A pinch of salt and black pepper
- 1 red bell pepper, chopped
- 5 cups vegetable stock
- 15 ounces tomatoes, chopped
- 1 tablespoon cilantro, chopped

Directions:

1. Heat up a pot with the oil over medium-high heat, add the onion, celery, carrot and the bell pepper and sauté for 10 minutes.
2. Add the cauliflower and the other ingredients, toss, bring to a simmer and cook over medium heat for 25 minutes more.
3. Ladle the soup into bowls and serve.

Nutrition facts per serving: calories 210, fat 1, fiber 5, carbs 14, protein 6

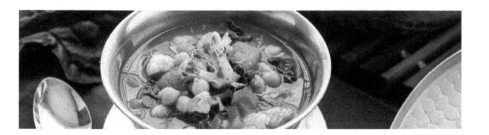

Lemon Cod Mix

Prep time: 10 minutes I **Cooking time:** 25 minutes I

Servings: 4

Ingredients:

- 4 cod fillets, skinless
- 2 garlic cloves, minced
- 2 shallots, chopped
- Salt and black pepper to the taste
- 2 tablespoons olive oil
- 2 tablespoons tarragon, chopped
- ½ cup black olives, pitted and halved
- Juice of 1 lemon
- ¼ cup chicken stock
- 1 tablespoon chives, chopped

Directions:

1. Heat up a pan with the oil over medium-high heat, add the shallots and the garlic and sauté for 5 minutes.
2. Add the fish and sear it for 2 minutes on each side.
3. Add the remaining ingredients, put the pan in the oven and cook at 360 degrees F for 15 minutes.

4. Divide the mix between plates and serve for lunch.

Nutrition facts per serving: calories 173, fat 3, fiber 4, carbs 9, protein 12

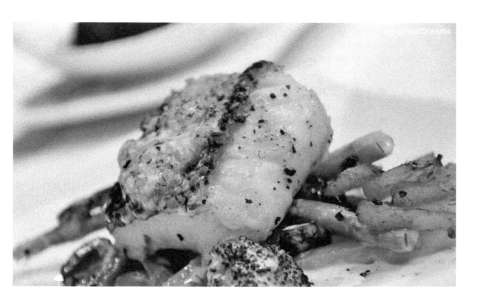

Kale and Lemon Soup

Prep time: 10 minutes I **Cooking time:** 15 minutes I

Servings: 4

Ingredients:

- 1 pound kale, chopped
- Salt and black pepper to the taste
- 5 cups vegetable stock
- 2 carrots, sliced
- 1 yellow onion, chopped
- 1 tablespoon olive oil
- 1 tablespoon parsley, chopped
- 1 tablespoon lemon juice

Directions:

1. Heat up a pot with the oil over medium heat add the carrots and the onion, stir and sauté for 5 minutes.
2. Add the kale and the other ingredients, toss bring to a simmer and cook over medium hea for 10 minutes more.
3. Ladle the soup into bowls and serve.

Nutrition facts per serving: calories 210, fat 7, fibe 2, carbs 10, protein 8

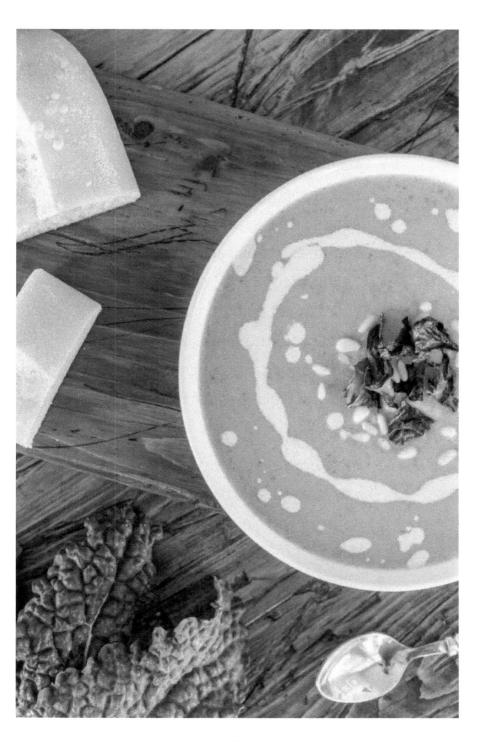

Balsamic Salmon Mix

Prep time: 10 minutes I **Cooking time:** 20 minutes I

Servings: 4

Ingredients:

- 4 salmon fillets, boneless
- 1 tablespoon olive oil
- 2 fennel bulbs, shredded
- 1 tablespoon balsamic vinegar
- 1 tablespoon lime juice
- ½ teaspoon cumin, ground
- ½ teaspoon oregano, dried
- 1 tablespoon chives, chopped
- Salt and black pepper to the taste

Directions:

1. Heat up a pan with the oil over medium heat add the fennel, stir and sauté for 5 minutes.
2. Add the fish and sear it for 2 minutes on each side.
3. Add the remaining ingredients, cook everything for 10 minutes more, divide between plates and serve.

Nutrition facts per serving: calories 200, fat 2, fiber 4, carbs 10, protein 8

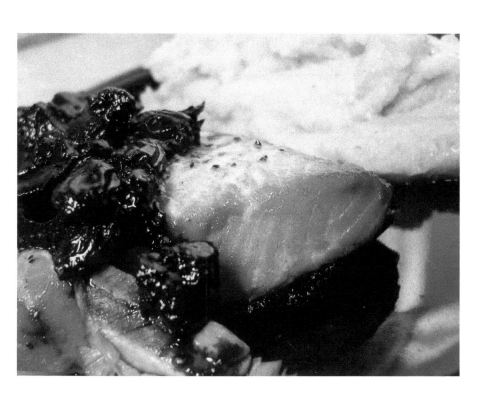

Turmeric Carrot Soup

Prep time: 10 minutes I **Cooking time:** 25 minutes I

Servings: 4

Ingredients:

- 1 pound carrots, peeled and sliced
- 2 tablespoons olive oil
- 1 yellow onion, chopped
- 1 teaspoon rosemary, dried
- 1 teaspoon cumin, ground
- 2 garlic cloves, minced
- A pinch of salt and black pepper
- 5 cups vegetable stock
- ½ teaspoon turmeric powder
- 1 cup coconut milk
- 1 tablespoon chives, chopped

Directions:

1. Heat up a pot with the oil over medium heat, add the onion and the garlic and sauté for 5 minutes.
2. Add the carrots, the stock and the other ingredients except the chives, stir, bring to a simmer and cook over medium heat for 20 minutes more.

3. Divide the soup into bowls, sprinkle the chives on top and serve for lunch.

Nutrition facts per serving: calories 210, fat 8, fiber 6, carbs 10, protein 7

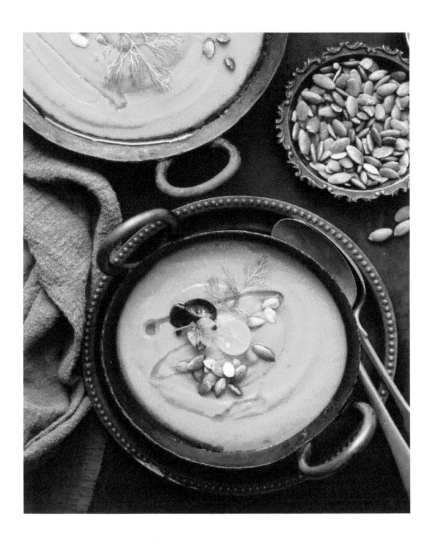

Coconut Leeks Soup

Prep time: 10 minutes I **Cooking time:** 20 minutes I

Servings: 4

Ingredients:

- 4 leeks, sliced
- 1 yellow onion, chopped
- 1 tablespoon avocado oil
- A pinch of salt and black pepper
- 2 garlic cloves, minced
- 4 cups vegetable soup
- ½ cup coconut milk
- ½ teaspoon nutmeg, ground
- ¼ teaspoon red pepper, crushed
- ½ teaspoon rosemary, dried
- 1 tablespoon parsley, chopped

Directions:

1. Heat up a pot with the oil over medium-high heat, add the onion and the garlic and sauté for 2 minutes.
2. Add the leeks, stir and sauté for 3 minutes more.
3. Add the stock and the rest of the ingredients except the parsley, bring to a simmer and cook over medium heat for 15 minutes more.

4. Blend the soup with an immersion blender, divide the soup into bowls, sprinkle the parsley on top and serve.

Nutrition facts per serving: calories 268, fat 11.8, fiber 4.5, carbs 37.4, protein 6.1

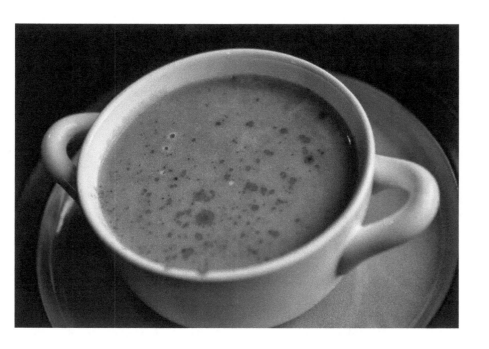

Paprika Turkey Mix

Prep time: 10 minutes I **Cooking time:** 40 minutes I

Servings: 4

Ingredients:

- 1 yellow onion, sliced
- 1 pound turkey breast, skinless, boneless an«
  roughly cubed
- 2 tablespoons olive oil
- Salt and black pepper to the taste
- 1 cup artichoke hearts, halved
- ½ teaspoon nutmeg, ground
- ½ teaspoon sweet paprika
- 1 teaspoon cumin, ground
- 1 tablespoon cilantro, chopped

Directions:

1. In a roasting pan, combine the turkey with th«
   onion, artichokes and the other ingredients
   toss and at 350 degrees F for 40 minutes.
2. Divide everything between plates and serve.

Nutrition facts per serving: calories 345, fat 12, fibe
3, carbs 12, protein 14

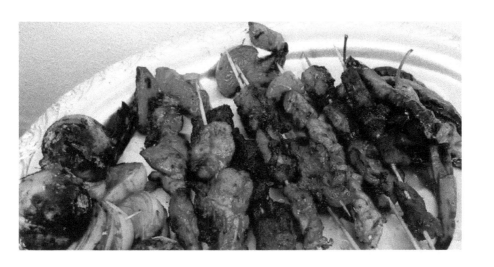

Salmon and Spinach Salad

Prep time: 10 minutes I **Cooking time:** 0 minutes I

Servings: 4

Ingredients:

- 2 cups smoked salmon, skinless, boneless and cut into strips
- 1 yellow onion, chopped
- 1 avocado, peeled, pitted and cubed
- 1 cup cherry tomatoes, halved
- 1 tablespoon olive oil
- 2 cups baby spinach
- A pinch of salt and cayenne pepper
- 1 tablespoon balsamic vinegar

Directions:

1. In a salad bowl, mix the salmon with the onion, the avocado and the other ingredients, toss, divide between plates and serve for lunch.

Nutrition facts per serving: calories 260, fat 2, fiber 8, carbs 17, protein 11

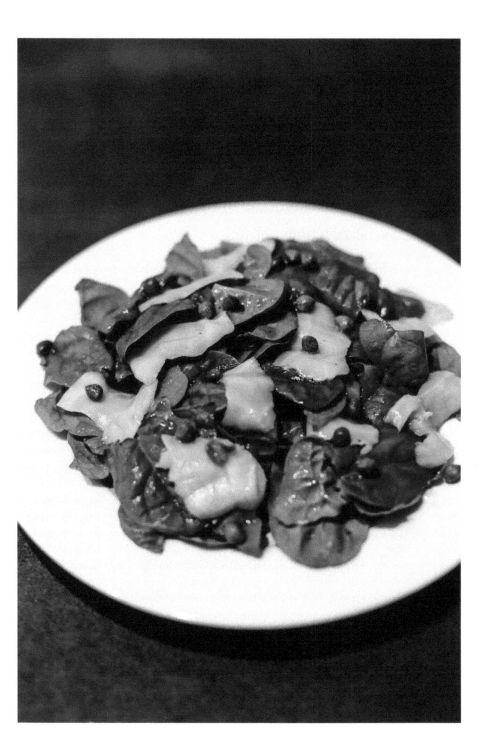

Turmeric Shrimp

Prep time: 10 minutes I **Cooking time:** 17 minutes I

Servings: 4

Ingredients:

- 1 pound shrimp, peeled and deveined
- 1 tablespoon lemon juice
- 2 zucchinis, sliced
- 1 yellow onion, roughly chopped
- 1 tablespoon olive oil
- 1 teaspoon turmeric powder
- A pinch of salt and black pepper
- 1 tablespoons capers, drained
- 2 tablespoons pine nuts

Directions:

1. Heat up a pan with the oil over medium-high heat, add the onion and the zucchini, stir and sauté for 5 minutes.
2. Add the shrimp and the other ingredients, toss cook everything for 12 minutes more, divide into bowls and serve for lunch.

Nutrition facts per serving: calories 162, fat 3, fiber 4, carbs 12, protein 7

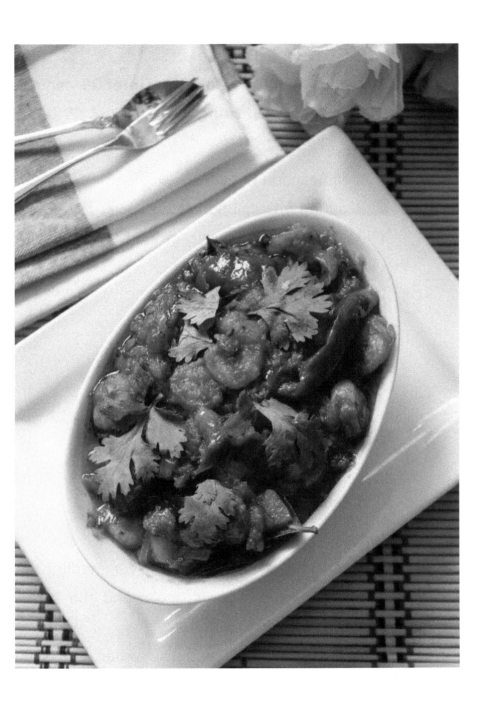

Broccoli Stew

Prep time: 10 minutes I **Cooking time:** 25 minutes I

Servings: 4

Ingredients:

- 1 tablespoon olive oil
- 1 pound broccoli florets
- ½ teaspoon coriander, ground
- 1 yellow onion, chopped
- 2 leeks, sliced
- 4 garlic cloves, minced
- ½ teaspoon turmeric powder
- A pinch of cayenne pepper
- 1 cup tomato paste
- A pinch of salt and black pepper
- 1 tablespoon lemon juice
- 1 tablespoon cilantro, chopped

Directions:

1. Heat up a pot with the oil over medium heat add the onion, garlic, leeks and the turmeric and sauté for 5 minutes.
2. Add the broccoli and the other ingredients toss, bring to a simmer and cook over medium heat for 25 minutes more.
3. Divide into bowls and serve for lunch.

Nutrition facts per serving: calories 113, fat 4.1, fiber 4.5, carbs 17.7, protein 4.4

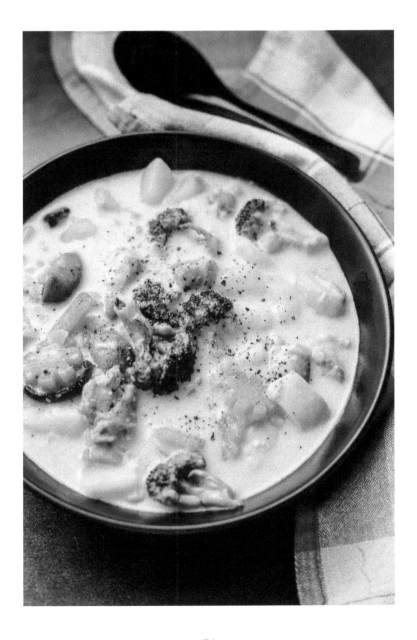

Salmon with Garlic Green Beans

Prep time: 10 minutes I **Cooking time:** 26 minutes I

Servings: 4

Ingredients:

- 2 tablespoons olive oil
- 1 yellow onion, chopped
- 4 salmon fillets, boneless
- 1 cup green beans, trimmed and halved
- 2 garlic cloves, minced
- ½ cup chicken stock
- 1 teaspoon chili powder
- 1 teaspoon sweet paprika
- A pinch of salt and black pepper
- 1 tablespoon cilantro, chopped

Directions:

1. Heat up a pan with the oil over medium heat, add onion, stir and sauté for 2 minutes.
2. Add the fish and sear it for 2 minutes on each side.
3. Add the rest of the ingredients, toss gently and bake everything at 360 degrees F for 20 minutes.
4. Divide everything between plates and serve for lunch.

Nutrition facts per serving: calories 322, fat 18.3, fiber 2, carbs 5.8, protein 35.7

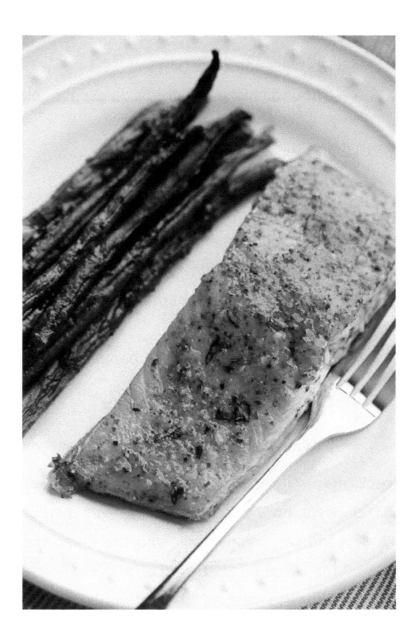

Coconut Chicken Stew

Prep time: 10 minutes I **Cooking time:** 45 minutes I

Servings: 4

Ingredients:

- 1 tablespoon olive oil
- 1 pound chicken thighs, skinless, boneless and cubed
- 2 garlic cloves, minced
- 1 small yellow onion, chopped
- 1 green bell pepper, chopped
- 1 red bell pepper, chopped
- ½ teaspoon cumin, ground
- ½ teaspoon sweet paprika
- 2 cups chicken stock
- A pinch of salt and black pepper
- 1 tablespoon lemon juice
- 1 cup coconut milk
- 1 tablespoon cilantro, chopped

Directions:

1. Heat up a pot with the oil over medium heat add the onion, garlic and the meat and browr for 10 minutes stirring often.
2. Add the rest of the ingredients except the coconut milk and the cilantro, stir, bring to a

simmer and cook over medium for 30 minutes more.

3. Add the coconut milk and the cilantro, stir, simmer the stew for 5 minutes more, divide into bowls and serve for lunch.

Nutrition facts per serving: calories 419, fat 26.8, fiber 2.7, carbs 10.7, protein 35.5

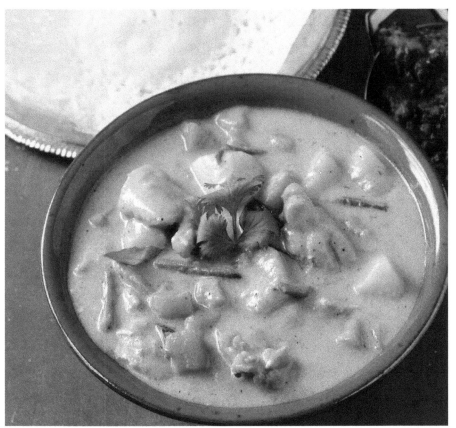

Lemon Turkey Stew

Prep time: 10 minutes I **Cooking time:** 45 minutes I

Servings: 6

Ingredients:

- 1 pound turkey breast, skinless, boneless an
  cubed
- 1 yellow onion, chopped
- 2 tablespoons olive oil
- ½ teaspoon mustard seeds
- 1 teaspoon ginger, grated
- 2 garlic cloves, minced
- 1 green chili pepper, chopped
- 1 teaspoon sweet paprika
- 1 teaspoon coriander, ground
- ½ teaspoon cardamom, ground
- ½ teaspoon turmeric powder
- A pinch of salt and black pepper
- 1 teaspoon lemon juice
- 1 cup chicken stock
- 1 tablespoon parsley, chopped

Directions:

1. Heat up a pot with the oil over medium-hig
   heat, add the onion, the meat, mustard seeds
   ginger, garlic, paprika, coriander, cardamor

and the turmeric, stir and brown for 10 minutes.

2. Add all the other ingredients, toss, simmer over medium heat for 35 minutes more, divide into bowls and serve.

Nutrition facts per serving: calories 202, fat 9.4, fiber 1.7, carbs 9.3, protein 20.3

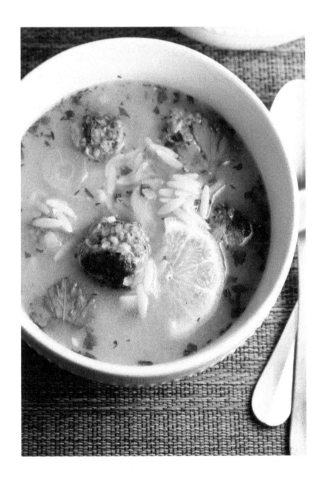

Salmon Pan

Prep time: 10 minutes I **Cooking time:** 25 minutes I

Servings: 4

Ingredients:

- 1 cup black beans, cooked
- 4 garlic cloves, minced
- 1 yellow onion, chopped
- 2 tablespoons olive oil
- 4 salmon fillets, boneless
- ½ teaspoon coriander, ground
- 1 teaspoon turmeric powder
- 2 tomatoes, cubed
- ½ cup chicken stock
- A pinch of salt and black pepper
- ½ teaspoon cumin seeds
- 1 tablespoon chives, chopped

Directions:

1. Heat up a pan with the oil over medium heat, add the onion and the garlic and sauté for 5 minutes.
2. Add the fish and sear it for 2 minutes on each side.
3. Add the beans and the other ingredients, toss gently and cook for 10 minutes more.

4. Divide the mix between plates and serve right away for lunch.

Nutrition facts per serving: calories 219, fat 8, fiber 8, carbs 12, protein 8

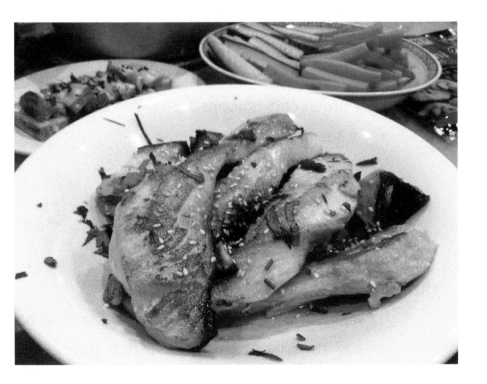

Cod Stew

Prep time: 5 minutes I **Cooking time:** 30 minutes I

Servings: 4

Ingredients:

- ½ pound cauliflower florets
- 1 pound cod fillets, boneless, skinless and cubed
- 1 tablespoons olive oil
- 1 yellow onion, chopped
- ½ teaspoon cumin seeds
- 1 green chili, chopped
- ¼ teaspoon turmeric powder
- 2 tomatoes chopped
- A pinch of salt and black pepper
- ½ cup chicken stock
- 1 tablespoon cilantro, chopped

Directions:

1. Heat up a pot with the oil over medium heat add the onion, chili, cumin and turmeric, sti and cook for 5 minutes.
2. Add the cauliflower, the fish and the othe ingredients, toss, bring to a simmer and cool over medium heat for 25 minutes more.
3. Divide the stew into bowls and serve.

Nutrition facts per serving: calories 281, fat 6, fiber 4, carbs 8, protein 12

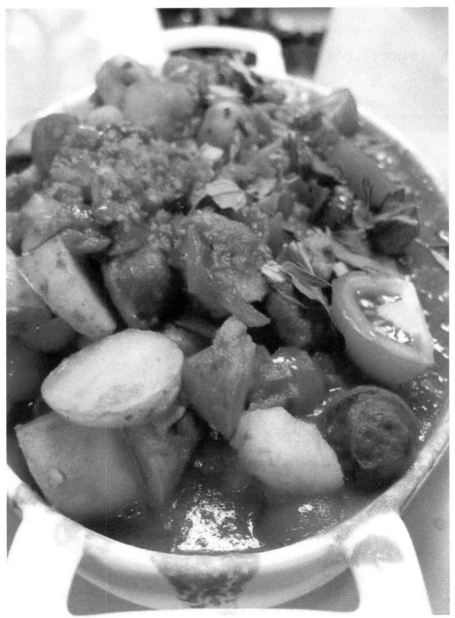

Cocoa Chicken Stew

Prep time: 10 minutes I **Cooking time:** 1 hour I

Servings: 6

Ingredients:

- 1 yellow onion, chopped
- 2 tablespoons olive oil
- 2 garlic cloves, minced
- 1 pound chicken breast, skinless, boneless an cubed
- 1 green bell pepper, chopped
- 2 cups chicken stock
- 1 tablespoon cocoa powder
- 2 tablespoons chili powder
- 1 teaspoon smoked paprika
- 1 cup tomatoes, chopped
- 1 tablespoon cilantro, chopped
- A pinch of salt and black pepper

Directions:

1. Heat up a pot with the oil over medium heat add the onion and the garlic and sauté for minutes.
2. Add the meat and brown it for 5 minutes more
3. Add the rest of the ingredients, toss, cook ove medium heat for 40 minutes.

4. Divide the chili into bowls and serve for lunch.

Nutrition facts per serving: calories 300, fat 2, fiber 10, carbs 15, protein 11

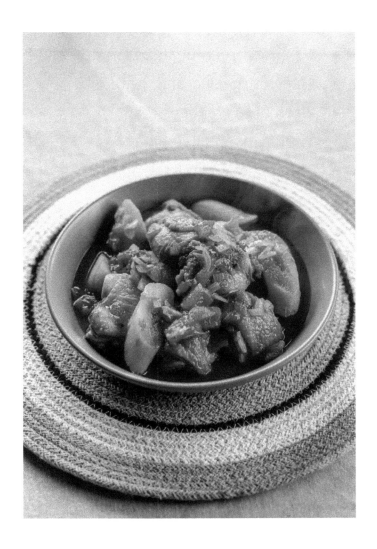

Chili Green Beans Soup

Prep time: 10 minutes I **Cooking time:** 35 minutes I

Servings: 6

Ingredients:

- 1 yellow onion, chopped
- 1 pound green beans, trimmed and halved
- 1 carrot, peeled and grated
- 2 tomatoes, cubed
- 1 tablespoon olive oil
- 2 teaspoons cumin, ground
- 6 cups veggie stock
- ¼ teaspoon chipotle chili powder
- 1 tablespoon cilantro, chopped

Directions:

1. Heat up a pot with the oil over medium heat, add the onion and the carrot and sauté for 5 minutes.
2. Add the green beans and the rest of the ingredients, toss, bring to a simmer and cook over medium heat for 30 minutes.
3. Ladle the soup into bowls and serve.

Nutrition facts per serving: calories 224, fat 2, fiber 12, carbs 10, protein 17

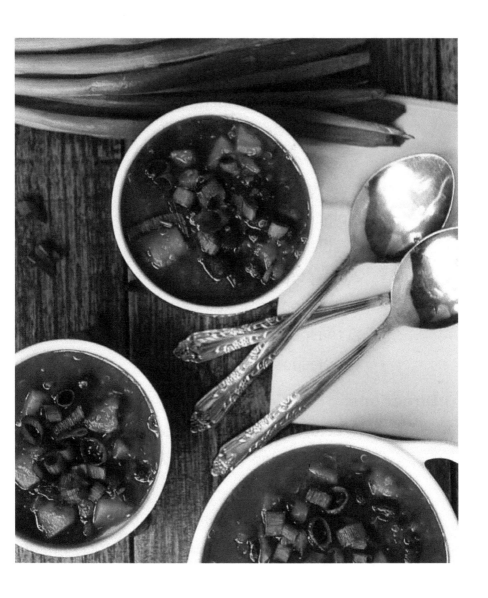

Cabbage and Carrot Soup

Prep time: 10 minutes I **Cooking time:** 35 minutes I

Servings: 6

Ingredients:

- 1 yellow onion, chopped
- 1 green cabbage head, shredded
- 2 tablespoons olive oil
- 5 cups veggie stock
- 1 carrot, peeled and grated
- A pinch of salt and black pepper
- 1 tablespoon cilantro, chopped
- 2 teaspoons thyme, chopped
- ½ teaspoon smoked paprika
- ½ teaspoon hot paprika
- 1 tablespoon lemon juice

Directions:

1. Heat up a pot with the oil over medium heat add the onion and the carrot and sauté for 5 minutes.
2. Add the cabbage and the other ingredients toss, simmer over medium heat for 30 minutes more, divide into bowls and serve.

Nutrition facts per serving: calories 212, fat 5, fiber 7, carbs 14, protein 12

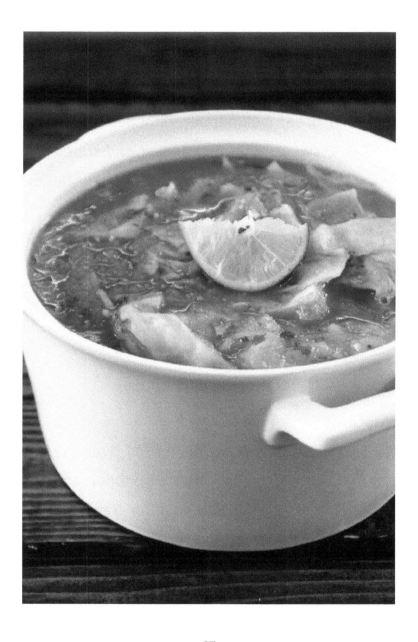

Turkey Soup

Prep time: 10 minutes I **Cooking time:** 45 minutes I
Servings: 4

Ingredients:

- 2 tablespoons olive oil
- 1 yellow onion, chopped
- 1 green bell pepper, chopped
- 2 sweet potatoes, peeled and cubed
- 1 pound turkey breast, skinless, boneless and cubed
- 1 teaspoon coriander, ground
- A pinch of salt and black pepper
- 1 teaspoon sweet paprika
- 6 cups chicken stock
- Juice of 1 lime
- A handful parsley, chopped

Directions:

1. Heat up a pot with the oil over medium heat, add the onion, the bell pepper and the sweet potatoes, stir and cook for 5 minutes.
2. Add the meat and brown for 5 minutes more.
3. Add the rest of the ingredients, toss, bring to a simmer and cook over medium heat for 35 minutes more.

4. Ladle the soup into bowls and serve.

Nutrition facts per serving: calories 203, fat 5, fiber 4, carbs 7, protein 8

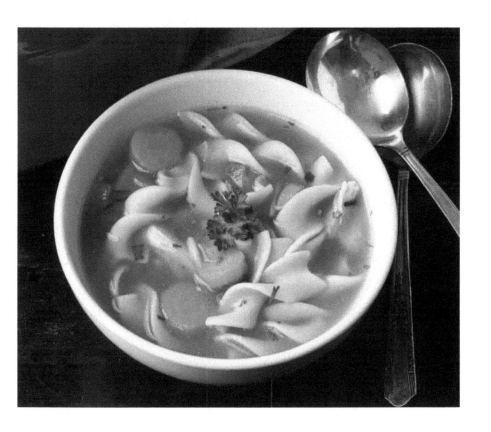

Beet Soup

Prep time: 10 minutes I **Cooking time:** 40 minutes I

Servings: 4

Ingredients:

- 2 tablespoons olive oil
- 1 yellow onion, chopped
- 2 beets, peeled and cut into large cubes
- 1 pound white mushrooms, sliced
- 2 garlic cloves, minced
- 1 tablespoon tomato paste
- 5 cups veggie stock
- 1 tablespoons parsley, chopped

Directions:

1. Heat up a pot with the oil over medium heat, add the onion and the garlic and sauté for 5 minutes.
2. Add the mushrooms, stir and sauté for 5 minutes more.
3. Add the beets and the other ingredients, bring to a simmer and cook over medium heat for 30 minutes more, stirring from time to time.
4. Ladle the soup into bowls and serve.

Nutrition facts per serving: calories 300, fat 5, fiber 9, carbs 8, protein 7

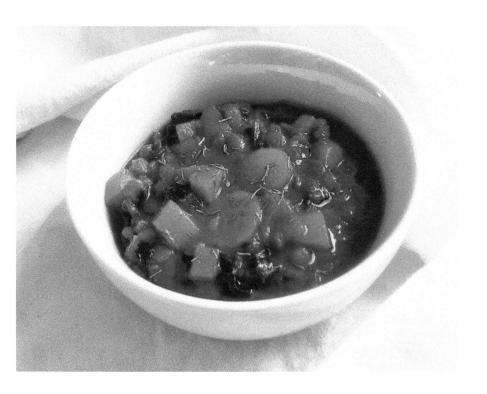

Meatball Soup

Prep time: 10 minutes I **Cooking time:** 30 minutes I

Servings: 4

Ingredients:

- 2 pounds chicken breast, skinless, boneless and minced
- 2 tablespoons cilantro, chopped
- 2 eggs, whisked
- 1 garlic clove, minced
- ¼ cup green onions, chopped
- 1 yellow onion, chopped
- 1 carrot, sliced
- 1 tablespoon olive oil
- 5 cups chicken stock
- 1 tablespoon parsley, chopped
- A pinch of salt and black pepper

Directions:

1. In a bowl, combine the meat with the eggs and the other ingredients except the oil, yellow onion, stock and the parsley, stir and shape medium meatballs out of this mix.
2. Heat up a pot with the oil over medium heat, add the yellow onion and the meatballs and brown for 5 minutes.

3. Add the remaining ingredients, toss, bring to a simmer and cook over medium heat for 25 minutes more.
4. Ladle the soup into bowls and serve.

Nutrition facts per serving: calories 200, fat 2, fiber 2, carbs 14, protein 12

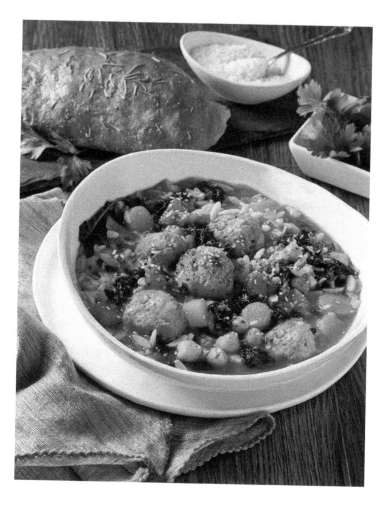

Chives Tuna

Prep time: 6 minutes I **Cooking time:** 18 minutes I
Servings: 4

Ingredients:

- 4 tuna steaks
- 1 tablespoon olive oil
- ½ teaspoon smoked paprika
- ¼ teaspoon black peppercorns, crushed
- Juice of 1 lemon
- 4 scallions, chopped
- 1 tablespoon chives, chopped

Directions:

1. Heat up a pan with the oil over medium-hig heat, add the scallions and sauté for 2 minutes
2. Add the tuna steaks and sear them for minutes on each side.
3. Add the remaining ingredients, toss gently introduce the pan in the oven and bake at 36 degrees F for 12 minutes.
4. Divide everything between plates and serve fo lunch.

Nutrition facts per serving: calories 324, fat 1, fibe 2, carbs 17, protein 22

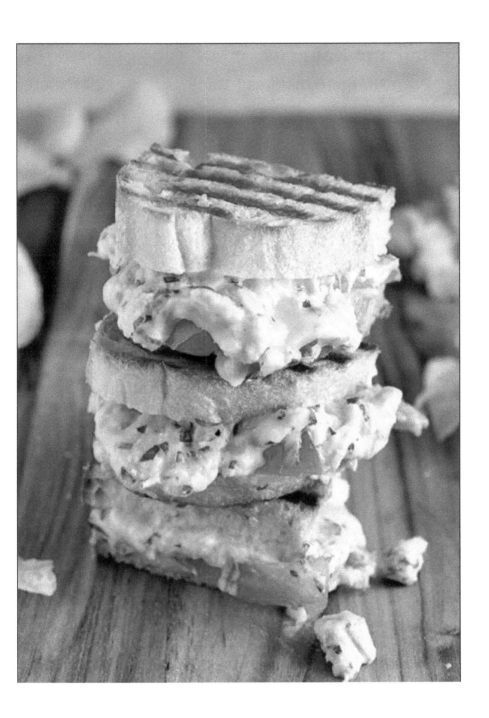

Fish and Kale Mix

Prep time: 10 minutes I **Cooking time:** 23 minutes I

Servings: 4

Ingredients:

- 4 sea bass fillets, boneless
- 2 scallions, chopped
- 2 garlic clove, minced
- 2 cups baby kale
- 2 tablespoons olive oil
- 1 tablespoon parsley, chopped
- Juice of ½ lemon

Directions:

1. Heat up a pan with the oil over medium heat, add the scallions and the garlic and sauté for 5 minutes.
2. Add the fish and sear it for 3 minutes on each side.
3. Add the rest of the ingredients, toss gently, cook everything for 12 minutes more, divide between plates and serve.

Nutrition facts per serving: calories 204, fat 9.8, fiber 0.8, carbs 3.6, protein 25

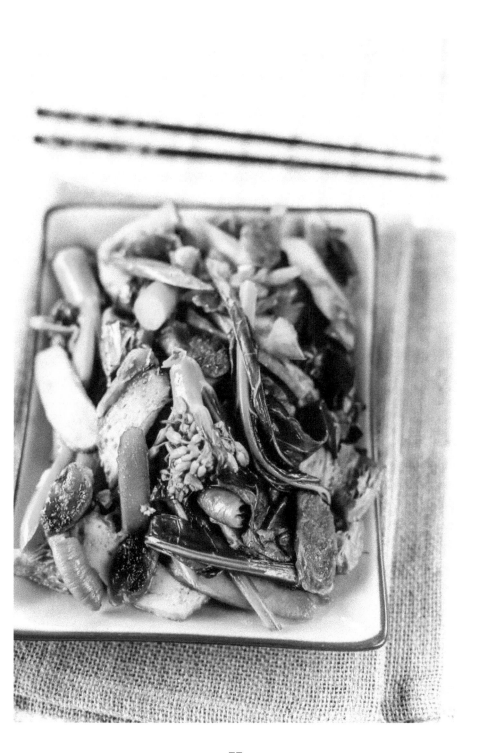

Chives Avocado Cream

Prep time: 10 minutes I **Cooking time:** 0 minutes I

Servings: 4

Ingredients:

- 3 avocados, pitted and peeled
- A pinch of salt and white pepper
- 1 yellow onion, peeled and chopped
- 3 cups water
- 2 scallions, chopped
- 1 tablespoon chives, chopped

Directions:

1. In your blender, combine the avocado with the onion and the other ingredients, pulse well divide into bowls and serve cold.

Nutrition facts per serving: calories 200, fat 12.3 fiber 7, carbs 13, protein 7

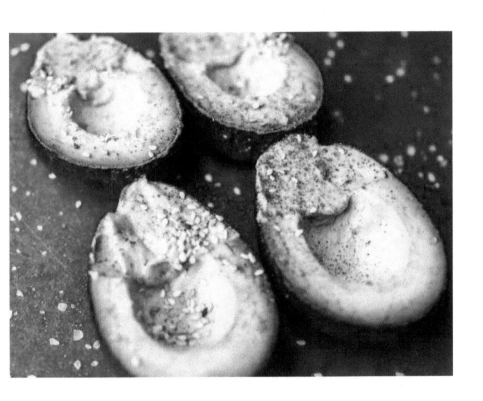

Coconut Asparagus Soup

Prep time: 10 minutes I **Cooking time:** 12 minutes I

Servings: 4

Ingredients:

- 1 yellow onion, chopped
- 1 bunch asparagus, trimmed and chopped
- 1 tablespoon olive oil
- A pinch of sea salt and white pepper
- 2 garlic cloves, peeled and chopped
- 2 cups almond milk
- ½ cup coconut cream

Directions:

1. Heat up a pot with the oil over medium heat add the onion and the asparagus and sauté fo 5 minutes.
2. Add the rest of the ingredients, toss, coo everything over medium heat for 7 minutes blend using an immersion blender, divide int bowls and serve.

Nutrition facts per serving: calories 191, fat 2, fibe 6, carbs 14, protein 7

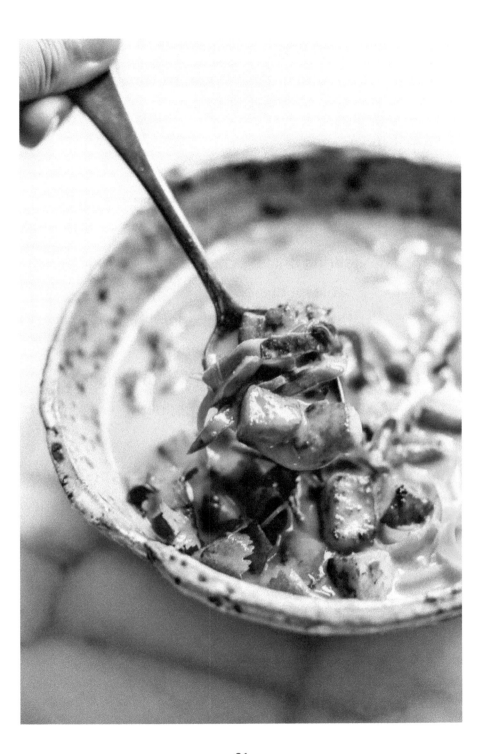

Basil Shrimp Mix

Prep time: 10 minutes I **Cooking time:** 12 minutes I

Servings: 4

Ingredients:

- 3 big tomatoes, cubed
- 1 pound shrimp, peeled and deveined
- 2 scallions, chopped
- 2 spring onions, chopped
- 2 tablespoons olive oil
- 1 tablespoon basil, chopped
- ½ teaspoon garlic powder
- A pinch of sea salt and white pepper
- 1 tablespoon chives, chopped

Directions:

1. Heat up a pan with the oil over medium heat, add the scallions and the spring onions, stir and sauté for 2 minutes.
2. Add the shrimp and the rest of the ingredients, toss, cook over medium heat for 10 minutes, divide into bowls and serve for lunch.

Nutrition facts per serving: calories 200, fat 4, fiber 6, carbs 14, protein 9

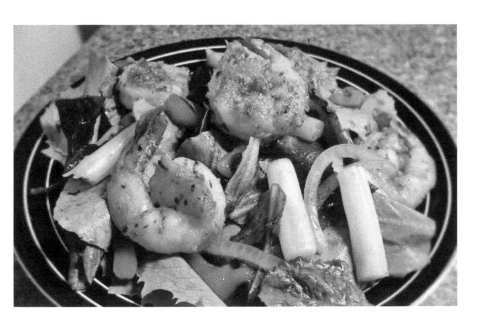

Salmon and Onion Pan

Prep time: 5 minutes I **Cooking time:** 16 minutes I

Servings: 4

Ingredients:

- 1 yellow onion, chopped
- 1 pound salmon fillets, boneless, skinless and cubed
- 1 tablespoon olive oil
- 1 tablespoon almonds, chopped
- A pinch of salt and white pepper
- ¼ cup chicken stock
- 1 tablespoon chives, chopped

Directions:

1. Heat up a pan with the oil over medium heat, add the onion and sauté for 2 minutes.
2. Add the salmon and cook it for 2 minutes on each side.
3. Add the rest of the ingredients, toss, cook everything for 10 minutes more.
4. Divide everything between plates and serve.

Nutrition facts per serving: calories 200, fat 11.3 fiber 0.8, carbs 3, protein 22.7

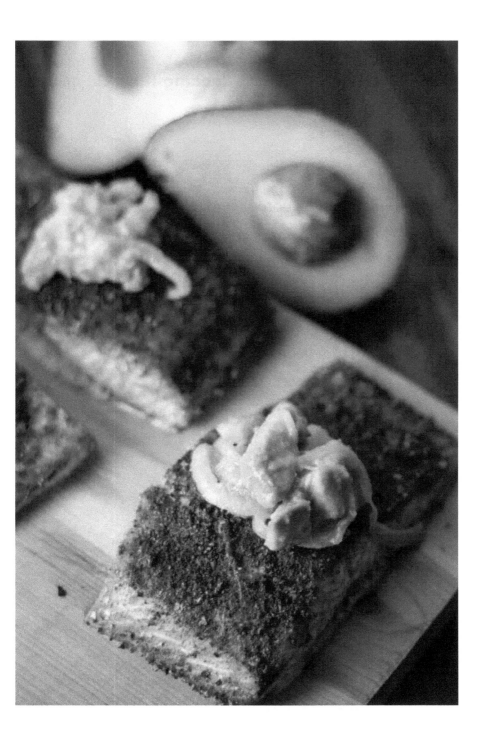

Mushroom and Garlic Stew

Prep time: 5 minutes I **Cooking time:** 30 minutes I

Servings: 4

Ingredients:

- 1 yellow onion, chopped
- 1 tablespoon olive oil
- 1 pound white mushrooms, sliced
- 1 cup chicken stock
- 1 cup tomato puree
- 1 carrot, sliced
- 1 teaspoon turmeric powder
- 1 teaspoon chili powder
- ½ teaspoon cumin, ground
- 1 teaspoon coriander, ground
- 2 garlic cloves, minced
- A pinch of salt and black pepper
- 1 tablespoon cilantro, chopped

Directions:

1. Heat up a pot with the oil over medium heat
   add the onion and the mushrooms, stir and
   sauté for 5 minutes.

2. Add the carrot and the garlic and cook for
   minutes more.

3. Add the stock and the other ingredients except the cilantro, stir, bring to a simmer and cook over medium heat for 20 minutes.
4. Divide the stew into bowls, sprinkle the cilantro on top and serve.

Nutrition facts per serving: calories 199, fat 4, fiber 6, carbs 14, protein 7

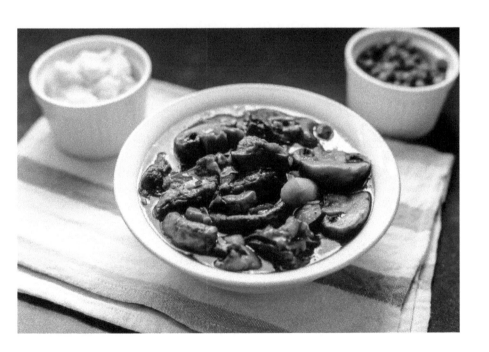

Green Beans and Cabbage Stew

Prep time: 10 minutes I **Cooking time:** 35 minutes I

Servings: 6

Ingredients:

- 2 tablespoons olive oil
- 1 yellow onion, chopped
- 2 garlic cloves, minced
- 1 tablespoon ginger, grated
- 1 red bell pepper, cut into strips
- 1 green bell pepper, cut into strips
- 1 cup cabbage, shredded
- 1 cup green beans, halved
- 1 cup tomatoes, cubed
- 2 zucchinis, sliced
- ½ teaspoon cinnamon powder
- A pinch of salt and cayenne pepper
- 3 tablespoons tomato paste
- 1 cup chicken stock
- 2 tablespoons lemon juice
- 1 cup kale, chopped
- 1 tablespoon cilantro, chopped

Directions:

1. Heat up a pot with the oil over medium heat, add the onion, garlic and the ginger, stir and sauté for 5 minutes.
2. Add the bell peppers and the other ingredients, toss, bring to a simmer everything, cook for 30 minutes more, divide into bowls and serve for lunch.

Nutrition facts per serving: calories 212, fat 7, fiber 7, carbs 12, protein 7

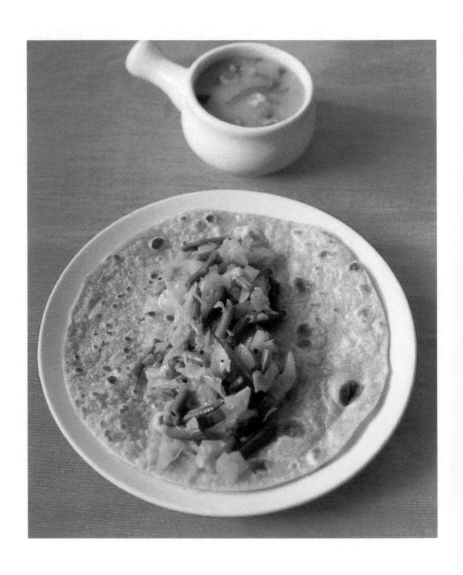

Shrimp and Pine Nuts Mix

Prep time: 10 minutes I **Cooking time:** 12 minutes I

Servings: 4

Ingredients:

- 2 tablespoons olive oil
- 4 scallions, chopped
- 1 pound shrimp, peeled and deveined
- 2 tablespoons pine nuts
- 1 yellow squash, peeled and cubed
- 2 garlic cloves, minced
- 2 tablespoons chives, chopped

Directions:

1. Heat up a pan with the oil over medium heat, add the scallions and the garlic and sauté for 2 minutes.
2. Add the shrimp and the other ingredients, toss, cook everything for 10 minutes more, divide into bowls and serve for lunch.

Nutrition facts per serving: calories 211, fat 6, fiber 4, carbs 11, protein 8

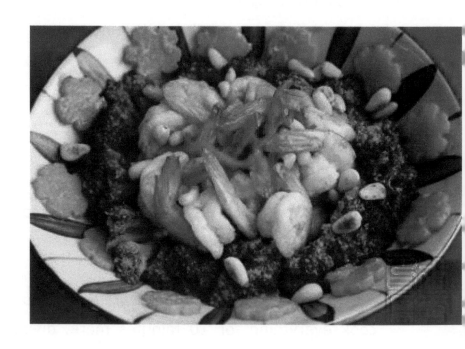

Quinoa Stew

Prep time: 10 minutes I **Cooking time:** 20 minutes I

Servings: 4

Ingredients:

- 1 tablespoon olive oil
- 1 yellow onion, chopped
- 2 garlic cloves, minced
- 1 cup quinoa, cooked
- 2 zucchinis, sliced
- 1 tablespoon ginger, grated
- 3 tablespoons coconut aminos
- 1 teaspoon chili powder
- 1 teaspoon cumin, ground
- 1 teaspoon turmeric powder
- 1 tablespoon hemp seeds

Directions:

1. Heat up a pan with the oil over medium heat, add the onion and the garlic and sauté for 5 minutes.
2. Add the quinoa, the zucchinis and the other ingredients, toss, cook everything for 15 minutes more, divide into bowls and serve for lunch.

Nutrition facts per serving: calories 182, fat 2, fiber 4, carbs 8, protein 11

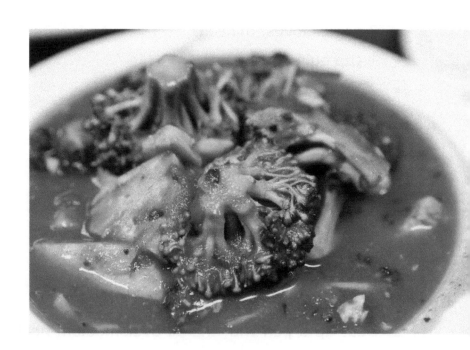

Chard Soup

Prep time: 10 minutes I **Cooking time:** 30 minutes I
Servings: 4

Ingredients:

- 1 yellow onion, chopped
- 2 tablespoons olive oil
- 2 garlic cloves, minced
- 1 pound chicken thighs, skinless, boneless and cubed
- ½ teaspoon turmeric powder
- ½ teaspoon red chili flakes
- A pinch of salt and black pepper
- 6 cups veggie stock
- 1 bunch chard, roughly chopped
- 1 tablespoon cilantro, chopped

Directions:

1. Heat up a pot with the oil over medium heat, add the onion and the garlic and sauté for 5 minutes.
2. Add the meat and brown for 5 minutes more.
3. Add the stock and the other ingredients, toss, bring to a simmer and cook over medium heat for 20 minutes more.
4. Divide the soup into bowls and serve.

Nutrition facts per serving: calories 181, fat 4, fiber 4, carbs 9, protein 11

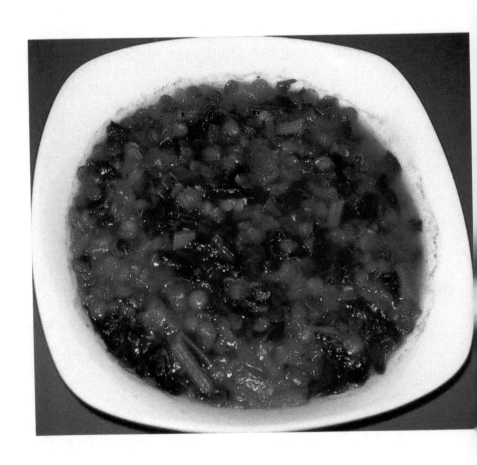

Salmon and Kale Salad

Prep time: 5 minutes I **Cooking time:** 20 minutes I

Servings: 4

Ingredients:

- 1 bunch kale, torn
- 4 scallions, chopped
- 2 garlic cloves, minced
- 1 tablespoon olive oil
- A pinch of salt and black pepper
- 1 cup peaches, cubed
- 1 pound salmon fillets, boneless and cut into strips
- 1 tablespoon pine nuts.
- 1 tablespoon lemon juice
- ½ tablespoon balsamic vinegar

Directions:

1. Heat up a pan with the oil over medium heat, add the scallions and the garlic and sauté for 2 minutes.
2. Add the salmon and cook for 5 minutes more.
3. Add the rest of the ingredients, toss gently, cook everything for 13 minutes more, divide into bowls and serve for lunch.

Nutrition facts per serving: calories 211, fat 4, fiber 8, carbs 16, protein 7

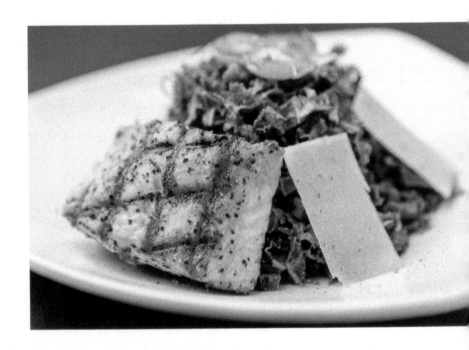

Sea Bass and Tomato Mix

Prep time: 5 minutes I **Cooking time:** 20 minutes I

Servings: 4

Ingredients:

- 4 sea bass fillets, boneless
- 1 yellow onion, chopped
- 2 tablespoons olive oil
- 1 tablespoon lemon juice
- 1 tablespoon oregano, chopped
- 2 garlic cloves, chopped
- Salt and black pepper to the taste
- 1 cup cherry tomatoes, halved
- 1 tablespoon chives, chopped

Directions:

1. Heat up a pan with the oil over medium heat, add the onion and the garlic and sauté for 2 minutes.
2. Add the fish and sear it for 2 minutes on each side.
3. Add the rest of the ingredients, cook everything for 14 minutes more, divide between plates and serve.

Nutrition facts per serving: calories 273, fat 6, fiber 6, carbs 10, protein 11

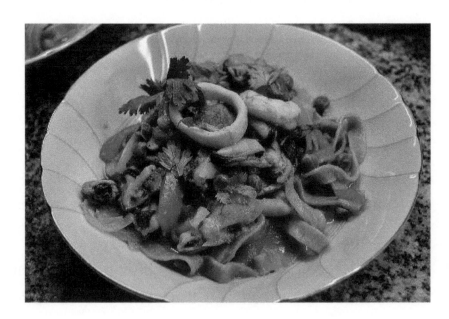

Paprika Salmon Mix

Prep time: 10 minutes I **Cooking time:** 15 minutes I
Servings: 4

Ingredients:

- 1 yellow onion, chopped
- 1 tablespoon olive oil
- 1 pound salmon fillets, boneless and cubed
- 2 teaspoons horseradish
- ¼ cup coconut cream
- A pinch of salt and black pepper
- ½ teaspoon sweet paprika
- 1 teaspoon cumin, ground
- 1 tablespoon chives, chopped

Directions:

1. Heat up a pan with the oil over medium heat, add the onion and the fish and cook for 5 minutes.

2. Add the rest of the ingredients, toss, cook everything for 10 minutes more, divide into bowls and serve for lunch.

Nutrition facts per serving: calories 233, fat 6, fiber 5, carbs 9, protein 9

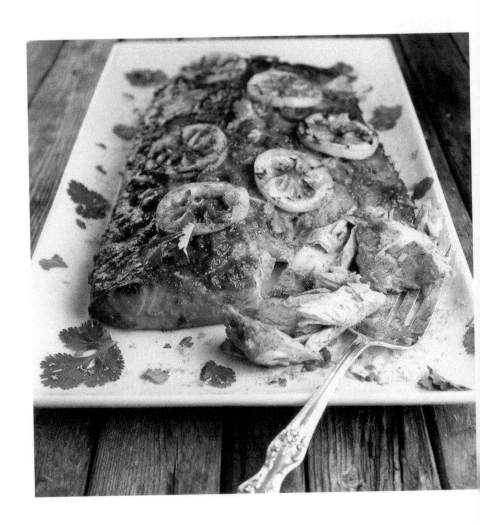

Cod and Capers Sauce

Prep time: 10 minutes I **Cooking time:** 15 minutes I

Servings: 4

Ingredients:

- 4 cod fillets, skinless
- 2 tablespoons mustard
- 1 tablespoon olive oil
- 4 scallions, chopped
- 1 tablespoon capers, drained
- A pinch of salt and black pepper
- 2 tablespoons lemon juice
- 2 tablespoons cilantro, chopped

Directions:

1. Heat up a pan with the oil over medium-high heat, add the scallions and the capers and sauté for 2 minutes.
2. Add the mustard and the other ingredients except the fish, whisk and cook for 3 minutes more.
3. Add the fish, cook the mix for 10 minutes, divide between plates and serve.

Nutrition facts per serving: calories 261, fat 8, fiber 1, carbs 8, protein 14

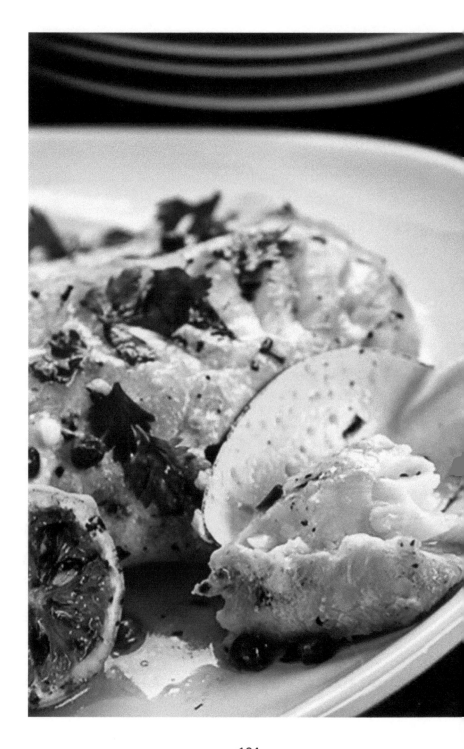

Salmon and Cucumber Salad

Prep time: 10 minutes I **Cooking time:** 0 minutes I

=Servings: 4

Ingredients:

- 1 pound smoked salmon, skinless, boneless and cut into strips
- 2 cucumbers, peeled and cubed
- 1 pineapple, peeled and cubed
- 1 tablespoon balsamic vinegar
- 2 tablespoons olive oil
- 1 tablespoon cilantro, chopped
- A pinch of salt and black pepper

Directions:

1. In a salad bowl, mix the salmon with the cucumbers, the pineapple and the other ingredients, toss and serve for lunch.

Nutrition facts per serving: calories 327, fat 12.2, fiber 1.4, carbs 10. 9, protein 21.9

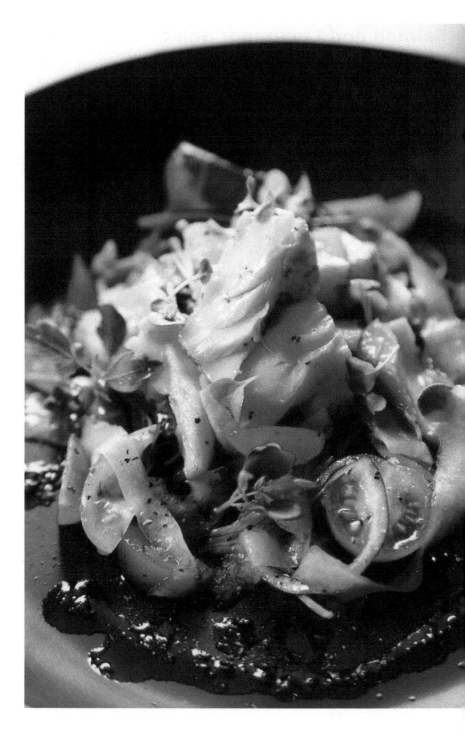

Citrus Salmon

Prep time: 10 minutes I **Cooking time:** 20 minutes I

Servings: 4

Ingredients:

- 4 salmon fillets, boneless
- 2 spring onions, chopped
- 2 oranges, peeled and cut into segments
- 2 tablespoons olive oil
- 1 cup walnuts, chopped
- 1 tablespoon chives, chopped
- A pinch of salt and black pepper

Directions:

1. Heat up a pan with the oil over medium heat, add the spring onions and the salmon and cook for 3 minutes on each side.
2. Add the rest of the ingredients, cook for 15 minutes more, divide between plates and serve.

Nutrition facts per serving: calories 210, fat 6.3, fiber 3, carbs 7, protein 22.2

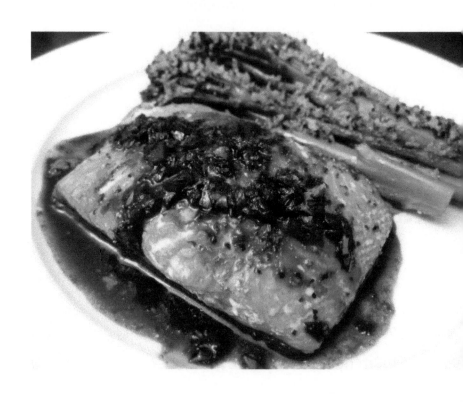

Chicken with Tomato Barley Mix

Prep time: 10 minutes I **Cooking time:** 25 minutes I

Servings: 4

Ingredients:

- 1 cup barley, cooked
- 1 pound chicken breast, skinless, boneless and cubed
- 1 tablespoon olive oil
- 3 scallions, chopped
- 2 tablespoons coconut aminos
- 1 tablespoon chives, chopped
- ½ cup tomato puree

Directions:

1. Heat up a pan with the oil over medium heat, add the scallions and the meat and brown for 5 minutes.
2. Add the barley and the other ingredients, toss, cook over medium heat for 20 minutes.
3. Divide everything between plates and serve for lunch.

Nutrition facts per serving: calories 231, fat 11, fiber 7, carbs 8, protein 9

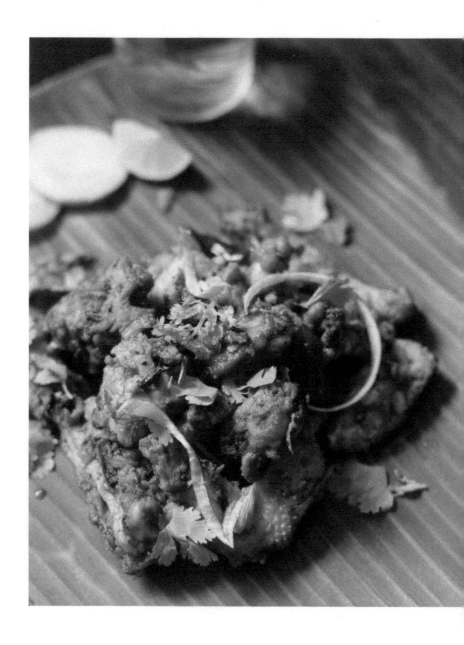

Lightning Source UK Ltd.
Milton Keynes UK
UKHW020635140621
385477UK00005B/127